Eyebrow Tinting Like A Professional

A quick and easy expert's guide

by

By Corinne Asch for MBA

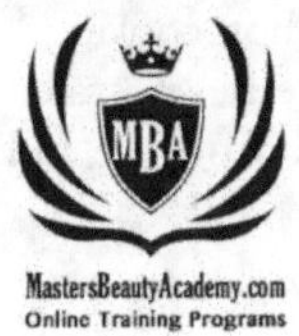

MastersBeautyAcademy.com
Online Training Programs

Published in U.S.A. by:
Create Space

© Copyright 2018 – Corinne Asch
ISBN 10 1729551246
ISBN 13 is 9781729551240

Table of Contents

Chapter 1

Benefits of Brow Tinting

Benefits of brow tinting

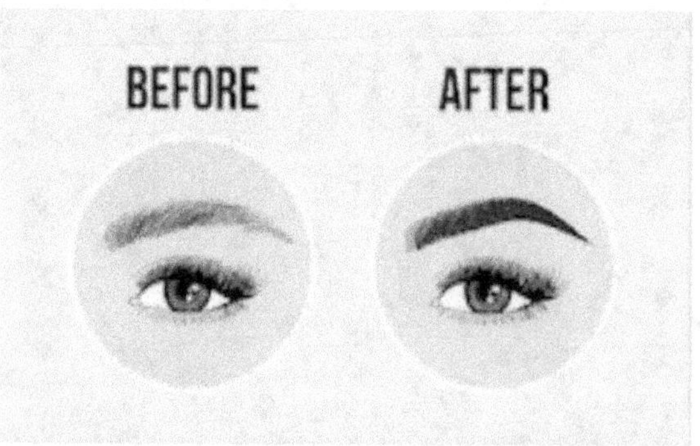

Brow tinting can not only benefit anyone with sparse or light eyebrows but even those lucky enough to have full brows.

Eyebrow tinting will have your brows looking naturally full, with a polished and put-together look!

Tinting our eyebrows is fun and so helpful in cutting down our getting-ready-time by taking away the need for any makeup (on the brows, anyway).

All my clients always get so many compliments for weeks after a brow tinting.

With eyebrow tint you will be able to create looks like Ombre brows, or powder brows.
It's really very easy!

You can switch it up and have Ombre brows one month and soft brows the next. You are only limited by your imagination.

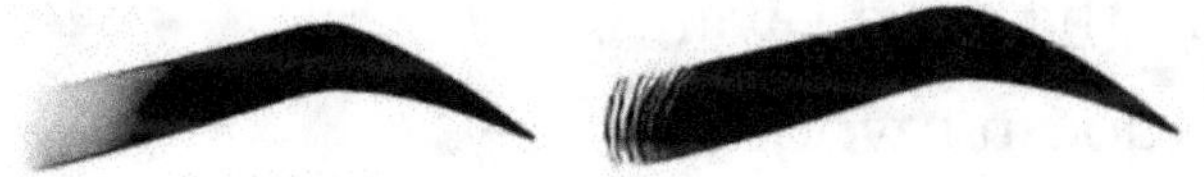

Getting your eyebrows tinted professionally would cost you anywhere from $25 to $50 **every month**. $600 a year.

Even if it didn't cost so much, who has time to add yet another appointment to their already busy schedules?

The truth is, this is a super easy procedure you can do yourself at home in 30 minutes or less.

Once you figure out your formula, you won't believe how simple this is and you will be doing a prettier job of it than any professional.

Don't make the mistake of seeing a pretty face with pretty brows and thinking 'those are the ones I want'.
It doesn't work that way.
You need to find the right brow shape for your face
How do you know which brows are the right ones for you?
One of my favorite ways is to find a celebrity that people tell you, you remind them of and see if you like her brows.

If you can't find a celebrity with brows you like then look around at people's faces and brows.

See if you can find someone with the same shape face as yours.
Look at her brows.

Another way is to look at the chart below, find your shape face and use the suggestions provided.

Chapter 2

Face Shapes And Their Brows

Face Shapes and Their Brow Shapes

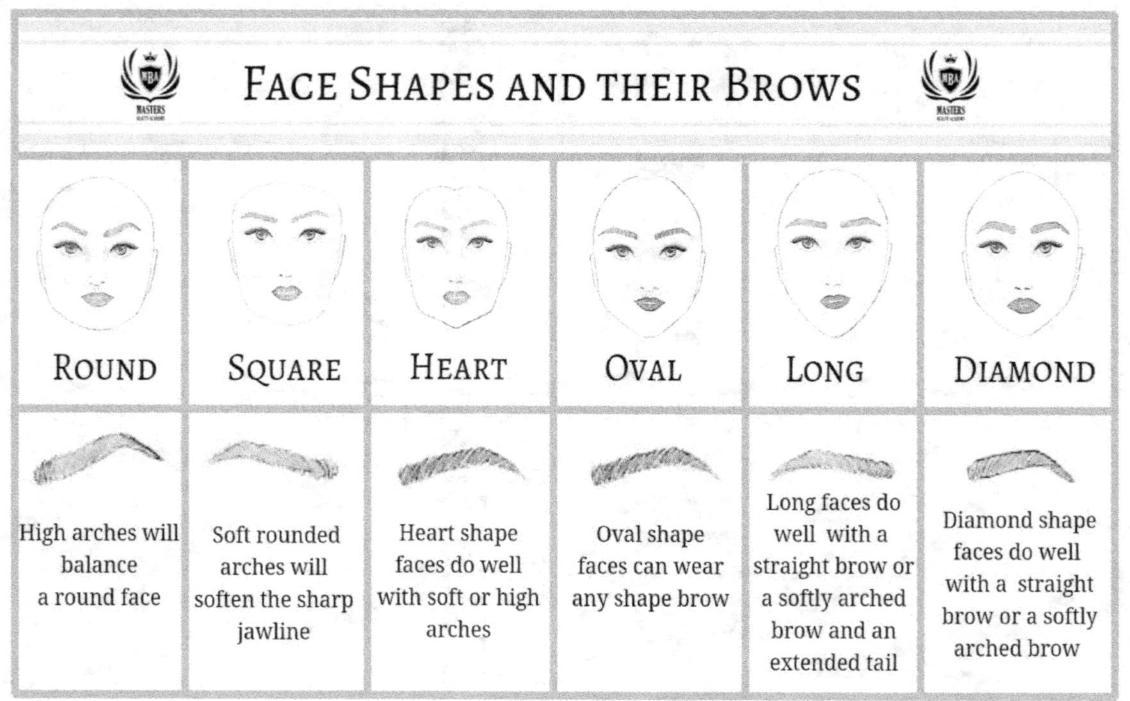

Round- Gigi Hadid, Selena Gomez, Queen Latifah, Renee Zellweger

* Face width and length are almost the same
* Widest at the cheeks

Goal: To make round face appear to be longer

Solution: A high arch eyebrow shape. Its up and down line would draw the viewer's eye up and down and lengthen it.
Avoid rounded brows as it makes the face more round.

Square- Jennifer Aniston, Paris Hilton, Nicole Ritchie, Demi Moore

* Forehead, cheekbones, and jawline are all almost the same width.
*Square and boney jawline is the prominent feature
Goal: To soften and balance the strong jawline.

Solution: Start with the curved eyebrow shape, then add more angle to create balance. The stronger and more bony the jawline is, the more angled the brow shape should be created.

A defined sharp peak at the top of the brow makes it appear longer.

Heart– Reese Witherspoon, Michelle Pfeiffer, Scarlett Johansson, Keri Washington

* Face strongly tapers towards chin
* Chin tends to be pointy
* Forehead may be a prominent feature

Goal: To soften and balance the strong pointy chin and the possibly prominent forehead.

Solution: Forehead may be the widest part of the face. Depending on how prominent the forehead is, start first with a low arch and round curved brows, then add more volume to it as it adds more length to the forehead as well as balancing the pointy chin.

Oval- Jessica Alba, Bella Hadid, Kate Middleton, Meghan Fox

* Face gracefully tapers toward chin
* Wider forehead
* Prominent check bones
Goal: To maintain this ideal oval face
Solution: A soft angled eyebrow shape would be best to maintain this ideal oval face but any this shape of face can wear any shape.

Long – Sarah Jessica Parker, Gisele Bundchen, Blake Lively, Jamie Lee Curtis

* Face gracefully taper towards the chin
* Elongated features from forehead to chin
* Some have a prominent chin
Goal: To make a long face appear shorter

Solution: A flat eyebrow shape is best for this shape face.

Its horizontal line would stop the viewer from seeing the elongated face, instead it makes it appear to be shorter. Elongate the tail of the brow so that it extends beyond the corner of the eye.

Diamond – Halle Berry, Cate Blanchett, Rihanna

* Face is very angular and somewhat bony
* Face is widest at temples
* Rarest face shape

Goal: To soften the whole face and to make the widest portion look less wide.

Solution: A curved eyebrow shape is best for this face shape. The curves will soften angled face and reduce the widest part of the face.

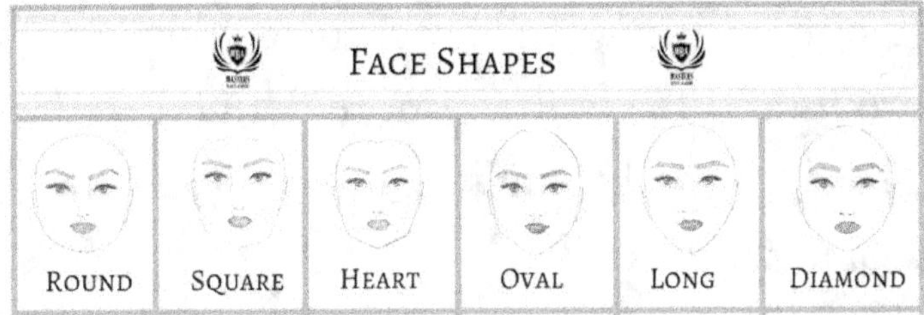

Note: Bringing the brows too close together will create a   masculine and authoritative look. This may be good for the male clientele. Spacing them a little further apart will make eyes that are too close together seem less so. A thin face does better with a slightly shorter brow, while a fuller face does better with longer brows.

What does all this have to do with eyebrow tinting?

Eyebrow tinting will accentuate your brows and make them more defined.
That is a good thing if you have good looking eyebrows.
So, make sure you have the right eyebrows before you accentuate them by tinting them.

Chapter 3

Choosing The Right Color

How to choose the right color

As a rule of thumb it is generally best to go a shade or 2 darker than your hair color.
This is a general rule.
In beauty, there are always exceptions to every rule.
Again, look at the celebrities, but this time, look at coloring.
What do you like best?
Dark hair with light brows? Be careful not to go too light and look like you have no eyebrows.

Interesting fact: *It was in fashion for women to shave off their eyebrows during the renaissance era.*
Did you know that Mona Lisa had no brows?
Don't believe me? Google it.

Darker brows- create a stronger more defined look.

Lighter brows- softens the look

Another rule is to stay away from any warmth in the color you will be using, even if you have a lot of warmth in your hair color.

The reason for this is that all color oxidizes (means it turns an odd shade of red in the sun and in certain lighting)

Eyebrows are even more partial to oxidization and often look and red in the sun. (Take notice of women's brows when you're outdoors).

For a more natural look, it is best to stay away from any warmth.

Let me explain what warmth is.

Warmth is any gold or red tones in hair color or dyes.

Keep the color neutral for the softest effect.

If you are so inclined, you could venture out and try adding a little gold to your formula and see what the outcome is.

Don't worry, eyebrow tinting only lasts

about 2 weeks.
If you love it you can use the formula forever.

Gold, reds and neutral are tones not color, so deciding on a tone does not give you a color.

The European colors usually come in numbers. They are made of the best ingredients and have the lowest amount of ammonia in them. (the EU is much stricter than the FDA).
Since the European colors have safer ingredients, we recommend you use European colors since we will be working so close to your eyes.
The American made brands are also numbers but each company has their own numbering system whereas the European ones all have the same system. These will be higher in ammonia (faster oxidization). The colors they produce generally don't last as long before oxidizing.

I personally recommend using the German brand called, Schwarzkopf Igora Royal brand which can be found on Amazon, *https://amzn.to/2QxlQJO*, but you can use any of the other European brands, such as Goldwell or Majirel for equally amazing results.

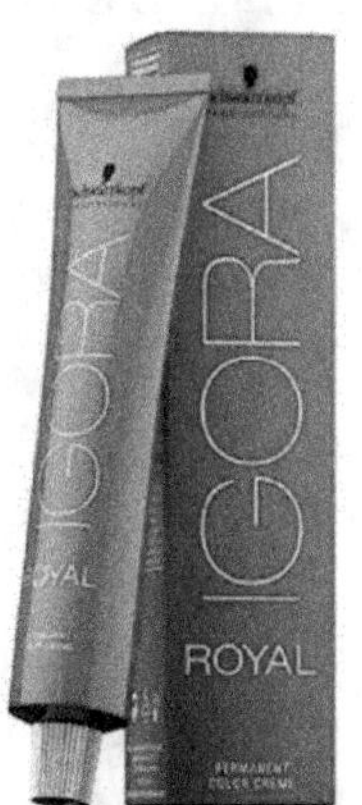

In European colors the numbers equal the colors and the numbers after the period equal the tones.

For example

1.0 = Neutral Black
1 is the darkest color
0 represents neutral (you will only ever see 0 after a period)

3.1 = Ashy Dark Brown
3 is a dark brown
1 after the period represents ashy tones

5.5 = Golden Medium Brown
5 is a medium brown
5 after the period represents gold tones

6.7 = Reddish Dark Blonde
6 is a dark blond
7 after the period represents red tones

8.0 = Light Neutral Blonde
8 is light blond
0 is neutral

10.5 = Lightest Golden Blonde
10 is the lightest color on the scale
5 after a period represents gold

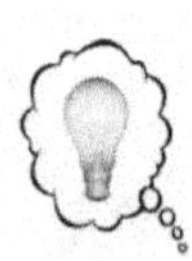

Colors are always darker than you would imagine them to be. Most people think of dark blond as being much lighter than it is. To the layman, dark

blond is a brown.

1 = Black
2 = Soft Black
3 = Darkest Brown   .0=Neutral
4 = Soft Dark Brown   .1 = Ash
5 = Light Brown   .4 = Beige
6 = Dark Blonde   .5 = Gold
7 = Medium Blonde   .7 = Copper
8 = Light Blonde   .8 = Red
9 = Lightest Blonde
10 = Ultra Blonde

On the next page you will find the Igora
color chart. There are way more colors
than you will ever need for your brows, but
it is to give you a chart where you can look
up your intended colors.

Colors can only lift a shade or two.
If you try to lift a color too high you will get
a brassy (unsightly red tones) color.

Starting color + added color = Outcome

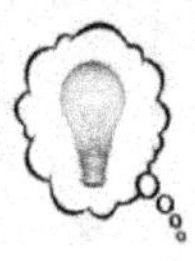

These color rules apply to hair as well

NATURALS · GOLDS · CHOCOLATES · REDS · HIGHLIFTS · SPECIALITIES · OPULESCENCE

Naturals & Golds

Level	NATURALS -0 NATURAL	-00 NATURAL EXTRA	-1 CENDRE	-11/-12/-13 CENDRÉ PLUS	GOLDS -4 ROSE	-5/-55 GOLD/GOLD EXTRA	-57 GOLD COPPER
9- EXTRA LIGHT BLONDE	9-0	9-00	9-1		9-4	9-55	
8- LIGHT BLONDE	8-0	8-00	8-1	8-11	8-4	8-55	
7- MEDIUM BLONDE	7-0	7-00	7-1		7-4	7-55	7-57
6- DARK BLONDE	6-0	6-00	6-1	6-12	6-4	6-5	
5- LIGHT BROWN	5-0	5-00	5-1		5-4	5-5	5-57
4- MEDIUM BROWN	4-0			4-13		4-5	
3- DARK BROWN	3-0						
1- BLACK	1-0		1-1				

Chocolates & Reds

Level	CHOCOLATES -6 CHOCOLATE	-63 CHOCOLATE MATT	-65 CHOCOLATE GOLD	-68 CHOCOLATE RED	REDS -7/-77 COPPER/COPPER EXTRA	-88 RED EXTRA	-98 VIOLET RED	-99 VIOLET EXTRA
9- EXTRA LIGHT BLONDE			9-65		9-7		9-98	
8- LIGHT BLONDE			8-65		8-77			
7- MEDIUM BLONDE			7-65		7-77			
6- DARK BLONDE	6-6	6-63	6-65	6-68	6-77	6-88		6-99
5- LIGHT BROWN	5-6	5-63	5-65	5-68	5-7	5-88		5-99
4- MEDIUM BROWN	4-6	4-63	4-65	4-68		4-88		4-99
3- DARK BROWN			3-65	3-68				
1- BLACK								

Highlifts, Specialities & Opulescence

Level	HIGHLIFTS 10- ULTRA BLONDE	12- SPECIAL BLONDE	PASTELS (CREATIVE)	BOOSTERS (CREATIVE)	NEUTRALISERS (TECHNICAL)	EXTRACTS (TECHNICAL)	OPULESCENCE FASHION
9- EXTRA LIGHT BLONDE	10-0	12-0	9.5-1	0-55	0-11	D-0	9-57
8- LIGHT BLONDE	10-1	12-1		0-77	0-22	E-0	8-19
7- MEDIUM BLONDE	10-14	12-11		0-88	0-33	E-1	7-48
6- DARK BLONDE		12-19	9.5-22	0-89			6-19
5- LIGHT BROWN	10-21	12-2	9.5-4	0-99			5-87
4- MEDIUM BROWN	10-4	12-4	9.5-49				
3- DARK BROWN	10-46	12-46					3-19
1- BLACK							

IV - IGORA VIBRANCE // IEM - IGORA EXPERT MOUSSE

Chapter 4

Mixing The Colors

Mixing Color

All colors are mixed 50% color and 50% peroxide, no matter what volume you use. To make sure you understand, it is equal parts color to peroxide.

You can measure at first to get an idea of the measurements, but you'll soon know exactly how much to put of each without measuring.

You'll be surprised by how little you need to do a set of eyebrows.

Use a little less than the size of a miniature marshmallow, add the peroxide and mix very well until all color is completely incorporated into the peroxide.

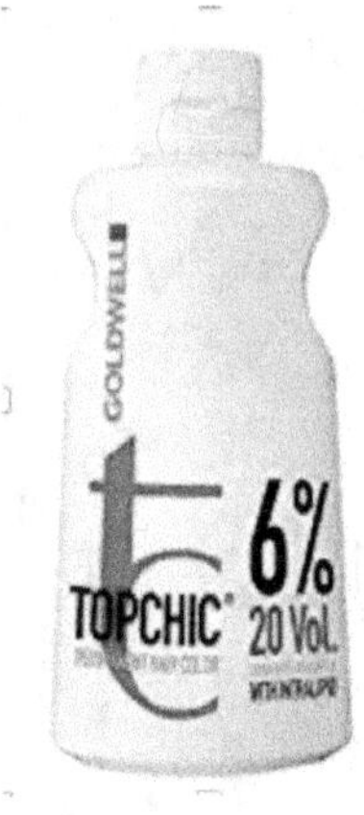

Which peroxide you use matters. Use a crème peroxide and not the much harsher watery version. Plus, we don't want the color to run so a crème peroxide makes the most sense. Peroxide comes in 10, 20, 30, and 40 volume. (Peroxide also comes in 130 volume, but that's for Balleyage and doesn't concern us here.)

If you are looking to make your brows darker, 10 volume peroxide will be the choice. At 10% volume, the color will deposit only. No lift.

If you are looking to lift and deposit, such as if you have gray hairs in the brows or you would like to lighten the brow color a bit, you will be choosing 20 volume peroxide.

If you need more than one shade lifted, I recommend to pre-lighten using hair bleach first.

I recommend Quick Blue by L'Oreal http://bit.ly/2NtuHu8

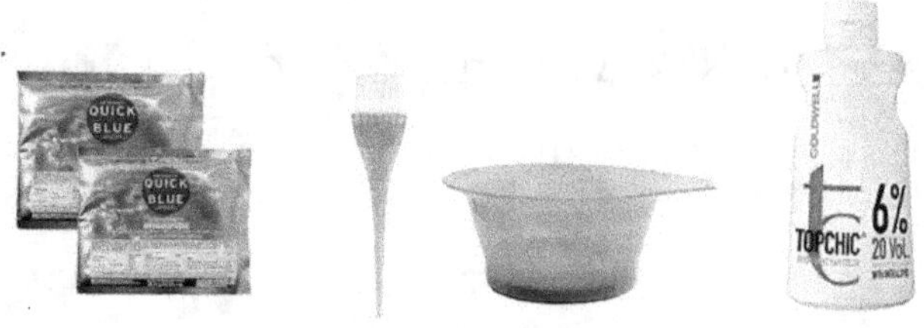

Mix 1 tsp of bleach with 10 volume of

peroxide if you are a natural level 6 or above and 20 volume peroxide if you are a natural level 5 or below.

Add enough peroxide to get the bleach the consistency of Greek yogurt.

To a thicker consistency add more of the powdered bleach.

To thin it out, add more peroxide.

Be sure to get your consistency thick enough not to run.

Apply the bleach to the brows and wait about 5 minutes.

Be careful not to let drip down. If need be, add a piece of cotton to the brow. The solution will hold it in place.

Check the color by using the back of a comb to scrape off the bleach. Look at the color. Is there a lot of red to it? Then re-apply and leave it on a little longer. Check again every 2 minutes until you reach the desired lift.

Don't look for the right color, that will rarely come from bleach and we will achieve that with color later.

You are only looking for the right level of lift.

Watch it carefully, bleach works fast. Don't let it get too light or the color will have trouble holding.

Wipe the bleach off with a Kleenex then wash off with soap and water being careful not to let the soap and water get in your eyes. Dry with a towel.

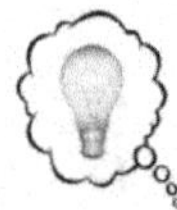

Apply color over bleached brows even if you like the color you got using bleach. Without the color, they will look unnatural in the daylight.

Chapter 5

Applying the Color

Applying the color

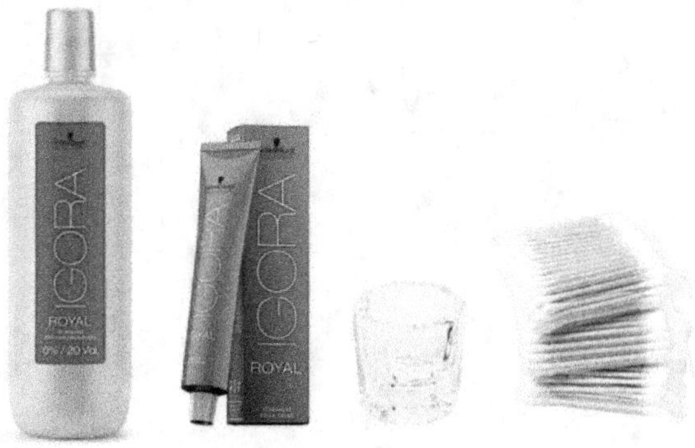

The first thing you will want to do is gently wash your brows to make sure there are no oils on the skin.

We want to make sure the skin grabs the color.

If you've bleached your brows or are darkening them and you don't have any gray hairs, you will be using 10 volume peroxide.

Everyone else will be using 20 volume,

which is the same volume used for hair color.

You've mixed your color well using a Q-tip or small wooden stick, like a match stick. Make sure the color and peroxide are completely mixed with no visible lumps.

Take your Q-tip or small eyebrow brush, dip into the color and pick up a generous amount. Carefully fill in your eyebrows trying your hardest not to go over the outline. Think of your coloring books when you were a kid. No going over the line.

If you do. Take a clean Q-tip and clean the outline so that the lines and the shapes are perfect.

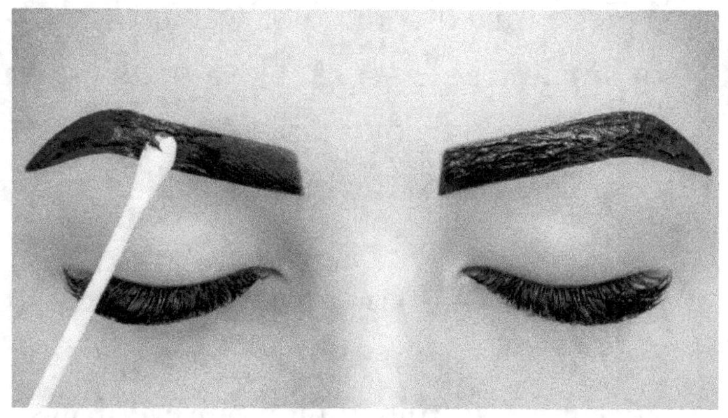

Apply a thick layer and let sit for no
more than 30 minutes.

Chapter 6

Ombre Brows

For Ombre brows-

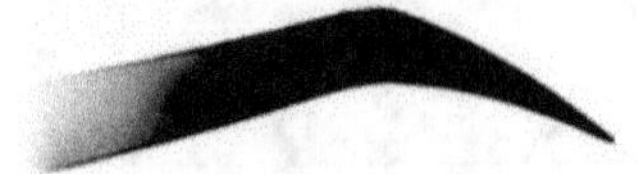

There are 2 ways to do Ombre

1. a)Apply color for ¾ of the brow and leave on for 20 minutes.
b.) Apply to the front of the brow for the last 10 minutes.

2. Apply your color to ¾ of the brow
a.) Mix a new color 1 shade lighter and apply to the front ¼ making sure to overlap with the back color.
b.) Leave color on brows for 30 minutes

Once color is ready to come off, wipe color off with a Kleenex, followed by a cotton pad soaked in make up remover or a gentle cleansing pad.
Wash your face and eyebrows gently. Let dry. Moisturize.

Chapter 7
Brow Color Formulas

Here are some formulas

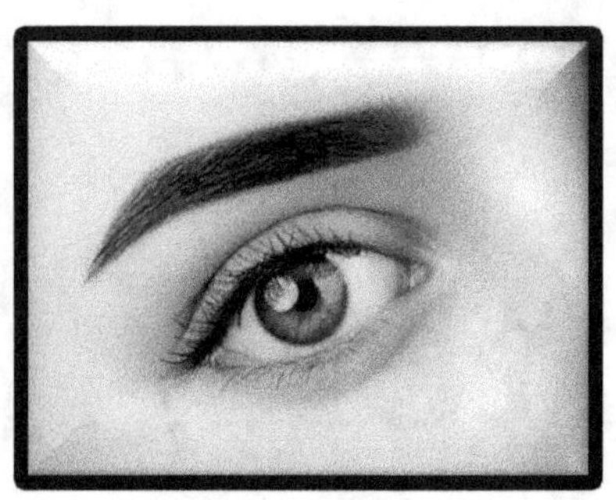

If you have dark brows 7.1+ 20 volume
If you have medium brows 6.1+20 volume
If you have light brows 5.0+ 10 volume

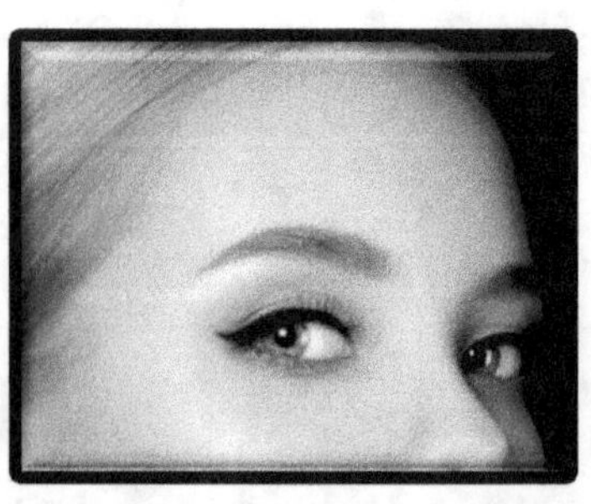

If you have dark or medium brown brows, you will need to pre-bleach then tone with 8.0 + 10 volume peroxide, if you got blonde from the bleach. If you got some red or too much gold you will be using 8.1 + 10 volume.

If you have medium or dark blonde brows you will use 7.1 + 20 Volume

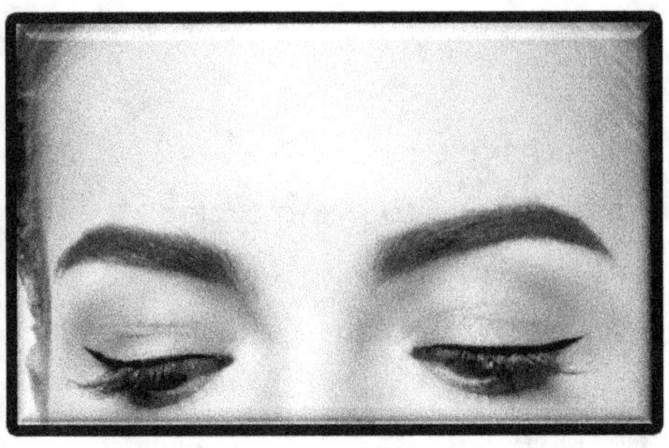

If you have dark brown brows you will use 6.1 + 20 volume
If you have medium brown brows use 6.1 + 20 volume

If you have light brown brows you will use 5.0 + 10 volume

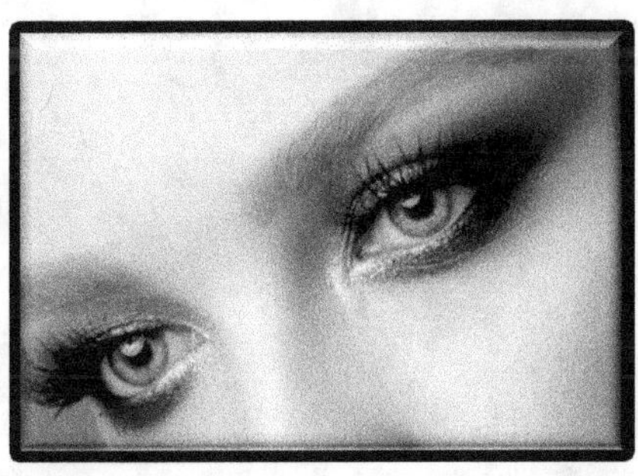

will need to pre-bleach your brows.
Once bleach you will tone the brows with 8.1 + 10 volume if you see any gold or red tones.

8.0 + 10 Volume if you eyebrows came up neutral.

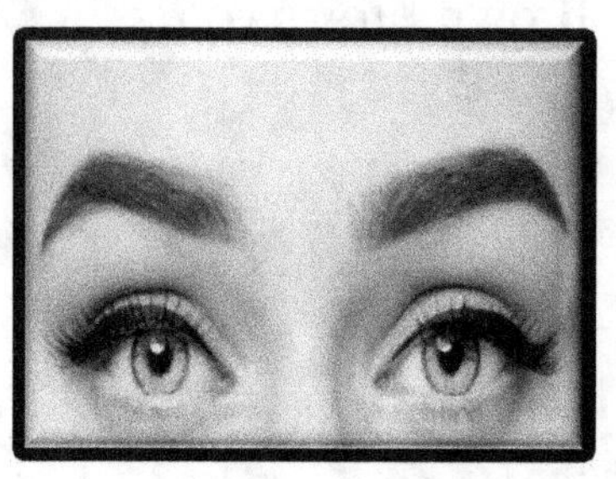

If you have dark brown brows
you will need to pre-bleach
and tone with 7.1 + 10
volume if you have a lot of
warmth.
7.0 + 10 volume if you got a
neutral color with the bleach
If you have medium brown brows you will use 7.1 + 20
volume. If you have light brows you will use 7.0 + 10
volume.

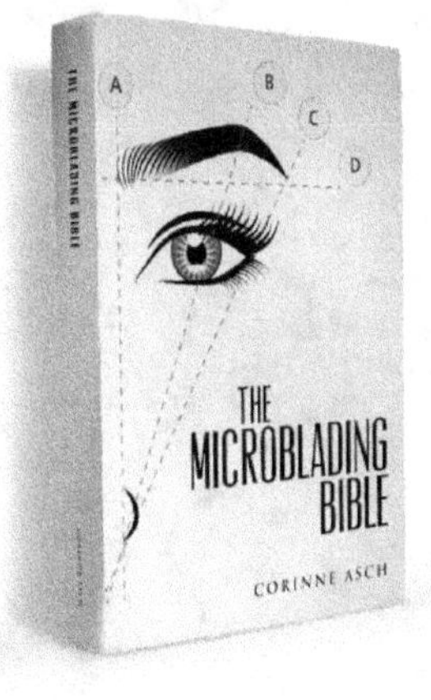

Corinne Asch is also the author of the best selling microblading book, <u>The Microblading Bible</u>

You can also find Corinne on <u>Facebook</u> And <u>Pinterest</u>

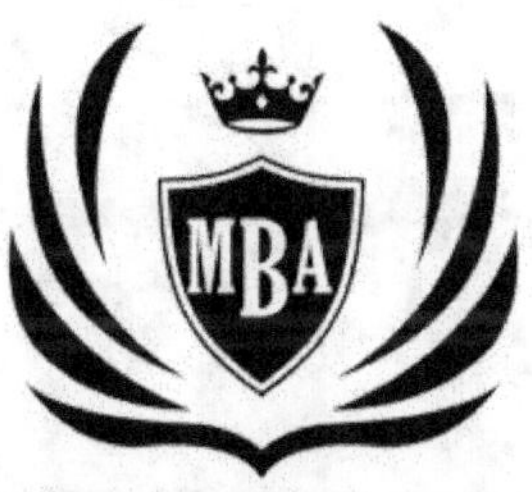

For the best Microblading online training and certification go to:

Masters Beauty Academy
Online Training Programs